What you really need to know about

HIGH BLOOD PRESSURE

Dr. Robert Buckman

with Patsy Westcott

Introduced by John Cleese

Macmillan Canada

Toronto

A Marshall Edition
Conceived by Marshall Editions, The Orangery, 161 New Bond Street, London W1Y 9PA

Edited and designed by Axis Design, 8c Accommodation Road, London NW11 8ED
First published in the UK in 1999 by Marshall Publishing Ltd.

First published in Canada in 1999 by Macmillan Canada, an imprint of CDG Books Canada Inc.

Copyright © 1999 Marshall Editions Developments Ltd.
All rights reserved. The use of any part of this publication reproduced, transmitted in any form
or by any means, electronic, mechanical, recording or otherwise, or stored in a retrieval system,
without prior consent of the publisher is an infringement of the copyright law. In the case of
photocopying or other reprographic copying of the material, a licence must be obtained from the
Canadian Copyright Licensing Agency (CANCOPY) before proceeding.

Canadian Cataloguing in Publication Data
Buckman, Rob
What you really need to know about high blood pressure
Includes index
ISBN 0-7715-7667-6
1. Hypertension - Popular works. I.Cleese, John. II.Title. III.Title: High blood pressure.
RC685.H8B85 1999   616.1'32   C99-932340-7

Originated in Italy by Articolor. Printed in and bound in Italy by New Interlitho.

Managing Editor For Axis Design Jo Wells, Project Editor Theresa Reynolds, Indexer Susan Bosanko,
Art Editor Siân Keogh, Illustrator Kuo Kang Chen, Photographer David Jordan,
Managing Editor Anne Yelland, Managing Art Editor Helen Spencer,
Editorial Director Ellen Dupont, Art Director Dave Goodman, Editorial Coordinator Ros Highstead,
Production Nikki Ingram, Anna Pauletti, DTP Mike Grigoletti, Lesley Gilbert

This book is available at special discounts for bulk purchases by your group or organization for sales
promotions, premiums, fundraising and seminars. For details contact: CDG Books Canada,
99 Yorkville Avenue, Suite 400, Toronto, ON, M5R 3K5, Tel: 416-963-8830

The consultant for this book was Shari Leipzig M.D., who is an obstetrician and gynecologist in
general practice in New York City. She is also a clinical instructor of obstetrics and gynecology
at Mt. Sinai School of Medicine.

Authors and publisher have used their best efforts in preparing this book. CDG Books
Canada and the authors make no representations or warranties with respect to the accuracy
or completeness of the contents of this book and specifically disclaim any implied warranties
of merchantability or fitness for a particular purpose. There are no warranties that extend
beyond the descriptions contained in this paragraph. No warranty may be created or
extended by sales representatives or written sales material. The accuracy and completeness
of the information provided herein and the opinions stated herein are not guaranteed or
warranted to produce any specific results, and the advice and strategies contained herein
may not be suitable for every individual. Neither CDG Books Canada nor the authors shall be
liable for any loss of profit or any other commercial damages including but not limited to
special, incidental, consequential or other damages.

1 2 3 4 5 Marshall 03 02 01 00 99

Contents

Foreword

Most of you know me best as someone who makes people laugh.

But for 30 years I have also been involved with communicating information. And one particular area in which communication often breaks down is the doctor/patient relationship. We have all come across doctors who fail to communicate clearly, using complex medical terms when a simple explanation would do, and dismiss us with a "Come back in a month if you still feel unwell." Fortunately, I met Dr. Robert Buckman.

Rob is one of North America's leading experts on cancer, but far more importantly he is a doctor who believes that hiding behind medical jargon is unhelpful and unprofessional. He wants his patients to understand what is wrong with them, and spends many hours with them—and their families and close friends—making sure they understand everything. Together we created a series of videos, with the jargon-free title *Videos for Patients*. Their success has prompted us to write books that explore medical conditions in the same clear, simple terms.

This book is one of a series that will tell you all you need to know about your condition. It assumes nothing. If you have a helpful, honest, communicative doctor, you will find here the extra information that he or she simply may not have time to tell you. If you are less fortunate, this book will help to give you a much clearer picture of your situation.

More importantly—and this was a major factor in the success of the videos—you can access the information here again and again. Turn back, read over, until you really know what your doctor's diagnosis means.

In addition, because in the middle of a consultation, you may not think of everything you would like to ask your doctor, you can also use the book to help you formulate the questions you would like to discuss with him or her.

John Cleese

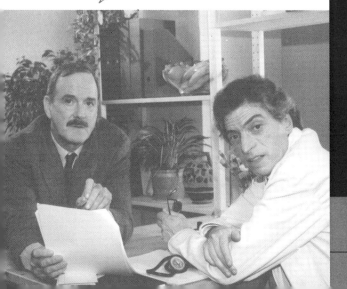

Introduction

The medical name for high blood pressure is hypertension.

The word means excessive tension in the circulatory system, not in the person.

High blood pressure is one of the most common conditions in the western world. It is thought that one adult in four has moderately raised blood pressure and around one in thirteen has it severely.

Although many people imagine high blood pressure to be a mild condition, left untreated it can lead to a number of serious medical problems. Research has shown that failure to control raised blood pressure is the leading cause for having a stroke. It also puts you at risk of angina or heart attack, heart failure, and kidney damage. In those people who have diabetes, it can be responsible for serious eyesight problems, which may result in blindness.

Your BP, as it is known in the medical profession, is the force exerted on the walls of the arteries as your heart pumps blood through the vast circulatory network of arteries, veins, and millions of capillaries.

In a healthy body the blood vessel walls are flexible and nothing impedes the blood flow as it constantly moves around the body delivering nutrient-rich oxygen to all the cells and carrying away the waste products to be eliminated. When the walls are adversely affected, and this could be for various reasons, they lose that essential elasticity. The heart has to work harder to make blood reach every part of the body.

Be aware

The trouble is that you won't necessarily know this since an increase in blood pressure causes no symptoms. You might think you'd get headaches or nosebleeds, but it isn't so. This is why it is vitally important for everyone to know what their blood pressure is by having it checked regularly so that, if it is raised, it can be medically treated with blood-pressure-lowering drugs.

Taking control

As research into heart and kidney disease has brought greater understanding of the importance of blood pressure, more is being done today to treat hypertension. You can be assured that if you have high blood pressure there are many simple, effective treatments that can be tailored to you as an individual.

As we all learn more about the effect of lifestyle on health, people with high blood pressure have a range of practical self-help steps they can take. The simplest rules are paying attention to what you eat and drink, quitting smoking, becoming more active, and avoiding stress. In mild cases these measures may even lower your blood pressure without the need for medication. Even if you do need blood pressure treatment, taking such steps can help increase the efficiency of treatment and give you a valuable sense of control.

Entering a partnership

Although it may be alarming to discover that you have high blood pressure, with treatment you have every chance of reducing it and increasing your chances of living a long, healthy life.

This book will tell you all you need to know about your blood pressure, how to find out if it is raised, and what can be done about it if you have a problem. With the information available in these pages you are able to enter a partnership with your doctor so you will know what questions to ask and when to ask them. A diagnosis of hypertension is a warning sign that you need to play a greater part in your own health to prevent the development of much more serious problems. This book will help you do just that.

Chapter

1

SYMPTOMS & DIAGNOSIS

How the heart works

At rest, your heart may beat 4,320 times and pump 275 quarts of blood an hour.

During activity, your heart may need to work five times harder than this.

A single blood cell can do a complete circuit of the body in about 45 seconds.

Your heart pumps blood through your blood vessels to supply every cell of your body with oxygen (from the lungs) and nutrients. With each beat your heart contracts, squeezing blood into the arteries and pumping it around your body. Blood is returned to the heart through the veins. The walls of the arteries are elastic, so they stretch slightly with each heartbeat to accommodate the surge of blood.

Tremendous force is needed to pump blood out of your heart and around your body. If you have high blood pressure the stress on the arteries is intense. As a result the smooth lining of the arteries becomes rough and their walls become thicker. Over time, this causes the arteries to narrow and become less elastic, a process known as arteriosclerosis or hardening of the arteries.

HOW BLOOD FLOWS AROUND THE BODY

Blood is pumped from the heart into the lungs where oxygen is added to it (this is called oxygenation). The oxygen-rich blood then returns to the heart, from where it is pumped to the brain and around the rest of the body, supplying oxygen to all of the cells. It returns, deoxygenated, to the heart, where the cycle begins again.

Heart

Body   Head

Lungs

Heart

WHAT DOES IT MEAN?

ANGIOTENSIN

A hormone normally present in the body that acts on the blood vessels and causes them to narrow.

ARTERIOLE

A medium-sized blood vessel that branches off an artery.

ARTERIOSCLEROSIS

Hardening and narrowing of the arteries. Can be a major factor in raising blood pressure above the norm.

RENIN

A hormone produced by the kidneys.

How blood pressure is regulated

Blood pressure is regulated by both the brain and the kidneys. The area of your brain that controls circulation receives messages about the level of blood pressure from pressure-sensitive nerves in the arteries. It responds by instructing smaller blood vessels called arterioles to narrow or widen as necessary. This alters the pressure in the arteries.

Blood pressure is also partly regulated by a hormone, called renin, produced by the kidneys. The production of renin causes the release of another blood chemical, angiotensin, which narrows the arterioles and raises blood pressure. Angiotensin also causes the adrenal gland to release a hormone that makes your kidneys retain too much salt. Salt increases the volume of blood in circulation, which causes blood pressure to rise.

YOU REALLY NEED TO KNOW

◆ The heart works like a pump, forcing blood around your body.

◆ Prolonged high blood pressure places great stress on the arteries.

◆ Over time, high blood pressure can lead to hardening and narrowing of the arteries.

◆ Blood pressure is regulated by control mechanisms in the brain and the kidneys.

How the heart works

What is blood pressure?

✓ You may have raised blood pressure without knowing it.

✗ High blood pressure is not an illness, although it is a risk factor for some conditions.

The heart pumps blood around the body through large blood vessels known as arteries, supplying your body and brain with oxygen and essential nutrients. The pressure of the blood traveling in the arteries is determined by how hard the heart works and the health of your blood vessels. High blood pressure, or hypertension as it is known medically, is when this pressure becomes too high.

What is normal?

It may sound odd, but "normal" blood pressure varies a lot. It varies from one person to the next, and in any individual it rises and falls naturally during the course of each day, depending on the workload of the heart. Moreover, everyone's blood pressure tends to rise slightly with age. Because of these differences, there is no set point at which high blood pressure is diagnosed. It depends on an individual's age and lifestyle.

HOW BLOOD PRESSURE CHANGES THROUGH A DAY

FOR MEN AND WOMEN

WHEN IT IS LOWER	WHEN IT IS HIGHER
◆ At night.	◆ During the day.
◆ When you are relaxing.	◆ With exercise or exertion.
◆ When you are asleep.	◆ While smoking a cigarette.
◆ When listening to quiet music.	◆ If anxious, stressed, or excited.
	◆ In cold weather.

LOW BLOOD PRESSURE

Low blood pressure, or hypotension as it is known, is not usually a medical problem. In fact, by and large if your blood pressure is low you are more likely to live a long, healthy life. Shock caused by a heart attack or heavy blood loss after an accident can cause a sudden and sometimes dangerous fall in blood pressure. In such cases, fainting may occur because the heart cannot sustain the blood supply to the brain; however, once the person is horizontal, blood flows back to the brain and consciousness returns. Occasionally, abnormally low blood pressure is a symptom of an illness that needs treatment.

In a normal, healthy young adult the average blood pressure measurement is around 120/80 (for an explanation of how blood pressure is measured, see p. 14). Ideally, your blood pressure should stay below 140/85. If, however, your blood pressure is consistently higher than this, and certainly if it rises above 160/90, you will need medical treatment.

Is high blood pressure a problem?

High blood pressure is not an illness in itself. In fact, most people who have it feel perfectly well and do not experience any symptoms. However, it is important that it is treated, because if it stays raised for any length of time it can damage the blood vessels and lead to serious health problems including eye problems, hardening of the arteries (arteriosclerosis), heart attack, stroke, heart failure, and kidney failure (see p. 24).

**YOU REALLY
NEED TO KNOW**

◆ High blood pressure can lead to a stroke, hardened arteries, heart attack, heart failure, and kidney failure.

◆ If your blood pressure is consistently raised you will probably need medical treatment.

◆ Only in rare cases does low blood pressure require treatment.

What is blood pressure?

13

Measuring blood pressure

It's easier to take your BP if you wear a sleeveless top or one with loose fitting sleeves that can be rolled up.

Try to relax your arm and breathe evenly when the nurse or doctor wraps the cuff around your arm.

Don't drink tea, coffee, or cola type drinks before having your blood pressure taken.

Don't smoke a cigarette or use a nicotine replacement patch one or two hours before your BP is measured.

There are high-tech machines available for measuring blood pressure, but it is most common for doctors and nurses to use a device called a sphygmomanometer, which is easier to use than it is to pronounce. It consists of a pump, an inflatable arm cuff, and a column of mercury in a glass tube. The pressure in the cuff causes the mercury column to rise up the tube: The height of the

HAVING YOUR BLOOD PRESSURE TAKEN

1. The cuff is placed around your upper arm and pumped up by the doctor or nurse, temporarily halting the blood flow. As a result your pulse can no longer be heard through a stethoscope placed against your arm.

2. As the cuff pressure is slowly released blood flow is restored and the doctor or nurse listens for a thumping noise as your heart contracts. This is the first measurement, the systolic.

3. As your heart relaxes between beats, the mercury column drops as the sound of blood flow becomes less distinct. When it disappears, the second measurement, the diastolic, is recorded.

BLOOD PRESSURE ON THE MOVE

Portable devices can be used to measure your blood pressure as you go about your daily activities. A printout tells your doctor your average blood pressure over the course of the day. This is known as ambulatory blood pressure monitoring (ABPM). It gives a more realistic idea of your blood pressure over time and often produces a lower reading than a single reading taken by the doctor.

column can be read in millimeters from the numbers printed on the tube. This is why blood pressure measurements are expressed in millimeters of mercury.

With each heartbeat, a pulse (surge) of blood is created in the arteries. The doctor or nurse can hear this pulse by placing a stethoscope on the brachial artery, which runs through your arm. This one is used because it is one of the major arteries branching from the aorta, the main artery leading from your heart; and also, being in the forearm, it is easily accessible, which means you don't have to get undressed.

The person taking your blood pressure listens for your pulse and notes the measurement at the point when your heart contracts and when it relaxes.

Sometimes the doctor may take two readings of your blood pressure: One while you are seated and another when you are standing. This is because blood pressure sometimes dips when you stand up (especially in older people). If your blood pressure is raised, the doctor may measure it a few times during your visit to the office to get an average reading.

YOU REALLY NEED TO KNOW

◆ Cutting off the blood flow with the inflatable cuff for such a short time isn't harmful.

◆ The doctor or nurse listens for the sound of your pulse in the main artery running through your arm.

◆ There are two measurements taken—one when the pulse begins again (the higher) and another when it fades or disappears (the lower).

◆ If the doctor thinks the readings taken in the office were too high you may be asked to use a portable device to check your BP at frequent intervals as you go about your everyday life.

Measuring blood pressure

Blood pressure readings

KNOW THE TERMS

✓ The actual point in the heartbeat cycle when the heart contracts is known as a systole.

✓ The point in the cycle when the heart relaxes is called the diastole.

✓ Hypertension is raised blood pressure. Hypotension is below "normal" blood pressure.

A blood pressure reading consists of two figures, written as 120/80 and read as "120 over 80." The upper figure is the measurement taken when your heart is contracting and is known as the systolic pressure. The lower figure is the one taken when your heart relaxes, and is known as the diastolic pressure.

Systolic pressure

The pressure in your blood vessels is at its peak when your heart contracts to squeeze blood into the arteries. This systolic pressure, measured when the doctor or nurse first hears the sound of your heartbeat, reflects the work of your heart and can vary a lot depending on what you are doing.

In a healthy person the systolic pressure is normally between 120 and 140 millimeters of mercury, written as 120 or 140 mm Hg (the chemical abbreviation for mercury.)

Diastolic pressure

The pressure in your blood vessels is at its lowest when your heart relaxes and fills with blood. This is known as the diastolic blood pressure, which the doctor or nurse

ISOLATED SYSTOLIC HYPERTENSION

Sometimes the diastolic blood pressure is normal but the systolic blood pressure is raised. Doctors call this isolated systolic hypertension (ISH). You are mostly likely to have it if you are over 65 and if you do the doctor will want to prescribe treatment because you could be at high risk of developing heart disease or having a stroke.

records at the last sound of your heart beating. In a healthy person the diastolic pressure is around 80 mm Hg. In general doctors prefer it not to go above 85, but 90 might be acceptable in some instances.

What the doctor is looking for

High blood pressure is diagnosed by looking at both the systolic and diastolic blood pressure. Usually if the systolic pressure is raised the diastolic pressure is too, and vice versa.

It used to be believed that raised diastolic pressure was more important than raised systolic pressure, because it is a sign that the medium-sized or small arteries have become stiff and narrowed. Research has now shown, however, that if you are over 40 years old a raised systolic pressure, which indicates how hard your heart is working, is also significant—especially in predicting whether you will develop heart disease.

Defining high blood pressure

There is no set measurement at which high blood pressure is treated. You may have borderline hypertension at 160/90 and treatment may depend on whether you have any other medical problems.

Your blood pressure is considered high if any of the following apply:

♦ the systolic pressure is 140 or higher.
♦ the diastolic is 90 or higher.
♦ both systolic and diastolic pressures are high.

The doctor will usually want to take appropriate action to reduce your blood pressure to the ideal target of 140/85 if you are otherwise well, or to a lower 130/80 if you have Type 2 (adult-onset) diabetes.

YOU REALLY NEED TO KNOW

♦ An average "normal" blood pressure reading is between 120/80 and 140/85.

♦ The upper figure (the systolic) reflects the way your heart is working. If you are over 40 years old it can predict the likelihood of heart disease.

♦ The lower figure (diastolic) measures the pressure in your arteries when your heart is at rest. If it is raised, it means your blood vessels are damaged.

Blood pressure readings

Self-monitoring

✓ Do consult your doctor before buying a self-monitoring device.

✓ Do make sure you are using a self-monitoring device correctly.

✗ Do not worry about a single high blood pressure reading—this can happen for all sorts of reasons.

Occasionally the doctor might suggest that you monitor your own blood pressure at home to provide information on how you are responding to medication, especially when it is first prescribed. It can also help the doctor to ascertain whether blood pressure lies behind other symptoms, such as light headedness. Self-monitoring can be especially useful if you need to have your blood pressure checked one or more times a day, or to keep an eye on it over a period of time.

Self-monitoring devices

You can buy electronic, non-mercury automatic or semi-automatic machines to take your blood pressure at home. Some, like the sphygmomanometer used at the doctor's office, measure the pressure in the brachial artery in your arm. Others measure the pressure by monitoring the pulse at your wrist (though this is not regarded as very reliable) or your finger.

Not all home monitoring devices are equally reliable. Seek your doctor's advice before buying one.

Using a self-monitoring device

If you do decide to use a self-monitoring device, follow the instructions carefully and ask your doctor or nurse for help if you are in any doubt about how to use it. Finally, remember that a single high blood pressure reading is unimportant. What matters is if your blood pressure is continually raised over a period of time.

To get an accurate long-term picture of your blood pressure, you should take the reading at a similar time each day and under similar conditions. To avoid a false high reading, choose a time when you are fairly relaxed. Resting for five minutes beforehand will help.

For best results, observe the following guidelines:

◆ Choose the same time of day to take your blood pressure, whether morning or evening.

◆ Wait half an hour after a cup of coffee or cigarette because caffeine and nicotine can cause a temporary rise in blood pressure.

◆ Sit comfortably and do a few minutes' calm breathing.

◆ Place the cuff or device on your arm or finger at heart level when you are taking the reading.

DEVICES TO MEASURE BP

There are two main types of device available. The automatic digital type, shown below, displays a reading on a small screen. The aneroid type, which is being used less and less because it is not very accurate, has a dial. For ease of comparison, the measurements produced by these devices are still expressed in millimeters of mercury even though mercury is not used in any of them.

YOU REALLY NEED TO KNOW

◆ There are no set figures at which high BP is diagnosed. It depends on age, lifestyle, and existing medical problems.

◆ Some people will need to keep a regular check on their blood pressure.

◆ It's important to follow your doctor's advice on how and when to do it, so you don't become over anxious.

Self-monitoring

Getting a diagnosis

SELF-HELP

✓ If you don't know what your BP is, make an appointment to have it taken.

✗ Anxiety can make your blood pressure rise, so try to relax before having it taken.

Because high blood pressure usually causes no symptoms the only way to find out if yours is normal or not is to have your blood pressure checked regularly. This is increasingly important as you get older, because blood pressure tends to rise with age.

The frequency of checks will vary depending on your health and your doctor's views. (Pregnant women, those taking the oral contraceptive pill, and diabetics are special cases; see Chapter 4.) If the doctor thinks you are at a high risk of developing high blood pressure because of your medical history, lifestyle, or other factors (see below), he or she may recommend more frequent checks.

HOW OFTEN SHOULD BLOOD PRESSURE BE CHECKED?

AGE	MEN	WOMEN
UP TO 35	Every five years provided you have no other health risks such as obesity.	Every five years provided you have no other health risks, are not pregnant, or taking the pill.
OVER 35	At least every two years or when you visit the doctor's office—whichever is first.	Every five years and ideally more often until menopause. After this, every two years or more frequently if using HRT.
DURING PREGNANCY		At every prenatal visit.
IF TAKING THE ORAL CONTRACEPTIVE PILL		Every six months.

FEAR OF DOCTORS

Anxiety can cause your blood pressure to shoot up, so it is important to be as relaxed as possible when you have your blood pressure taken. Some people's blood pressure goes up only when they see the doctor. This is known as "white coat" or "office" hypertension. Doctors do not yet know for certain the significance of this. It is known that many people become anxious when visiting the doctor for fear of a worrisome diagnosis, and this anxiety alone could cause blood pressure to rise. It is interesting, too, that some studies have shown that people with white coat hypertension are more likely to have an enlarged heart than those with normal blood pressure, and are more likely to need treatment for high blood pressure.

Ensuring an accurate picture

You won't be diagnosed as having high blood pressure because of the occasional high reading. The doctor will usually want to see at least three high readings on three separate visits over a period of a couple of months before making a firm diagnosis.

If your initial blood pressure reading seems unusually high, the doctor or nurse may take your blood pressure again after you have had a bit of time to relax. If your blood pressure still appears high, you may be asked to return to the office for further readings to be taken over the next month or so. Generally blood pressure settles down to the lowest level it is going to reach after around four visits to the office. This allows the doctor to decide if you need treatment.

YOU REALLY NEED TO KNOW

◆ Regular blood pressure checks are essential because high blood pressure causes no symptoms.

◆ The doctor won't make a diagnosis until there are three or four separate readings over a period of time.

◆ If you have "white coat" hypertension you may be asked to monitor your BP yourself at home.

Getting a diagnosis

Who gets high blood pressure?

SELF-HELP

Try to keep your weight within the ideal range for your height.

Learn some personal strategies for dealing with stress.

If you smoke, make a decision now to quit as soon as you can.

A diet with a lot of processed and junk food will not be healthy because of the high-fat, high-salt content.

It is not known exactly why some of us are more likely than others to develop high blood pressure but certain factors are known to increase the risk:

Race

Black Africans, African-Caribbean people living in Europe, and African-Americans have a higher risk. This may be partly related to the way the body handles salt.

Age

Our blood pressure rises fairly steadily between the ages of 20 and 40. After this it tends to increase more rapidly.

Sex

Women have slightly lower blood pressure than men during their 20s and 30s, but may develop BP elevation through hormonal changes, for example in pregnancy (see p. 64) or in using oral contraception. The same can also be true in older women using hormone replacement therapy (HRT) at menopause.

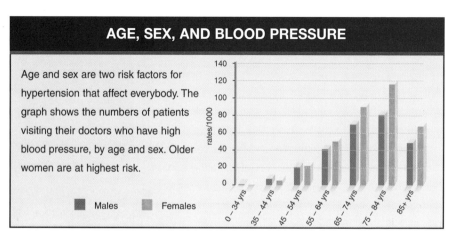

AGE, SEX, AND BLOOD PRESSURE

Age and sex are two risk factors for hypertension that affect everybody. The graph shows the numbers of patients visiting their doctors who have high blood pressure, by age and sex. Older women are at highest risk.

Males   Females

Family history

If one or both of your parents had high blood pressure you are twice as likely to develop it yourself.

Excess weight

Obesity is a significant risk factor for high blood pressure. Being overweight places strain on the heart.

Diet

A diet high in salt and fat and low in calcium, magnesium, and phosphorus has been linked to elevated BP. Avoid processed foods and eat more fresh fruit and vegetables. Eliminate salt from meals. Decrease alcohol consumption.

Stress

The role played by stress in the development of high BP is still uncertain. However, people whose blood pressure soars during stressful situations (the so-called "hot reactors") are more likely to go on to develop high blood pressure. Exercise relieves stress and can lower your BP.

Smoking

Smokers are more likely than non-smokers to develop high blood pressure; nicotine narrows the blood vessels.

Medical conditions

A number of illnesses, many of them hormonal disorders, are linked to hypertension.

Because of their medical condition, people with diabetes already have a higher risk of suffering stroke, heart, and kidney problems. The risk of these possible complications becomes even greater when high blood pressure is also a problem.

YOU REALLY NEED TO KNOW

◆ Some people are more prone than others to developing high blood pressure.

◆ Some of the factors that determine how likely you are to develop high blood pressure are out of your control. Others you can influence.

Who gets high blood pressure?

Effects on the body

SELF-HELP

✔ Make sure you have your eyes tested regularly.

✗ Don't ignore symptoms such as dizziness and headaches—see your doctor.

Some doctors call high blood pressure "the silent killer" because it stealthily damages the heart, blood vessels, kidneys, and other organs with few or no symptoms. In fact, about half of all people with high blood pressure are completely unaware of it. Occasionally, if blood pressure is exceptionally high, people may experience headaches, dizziness, and blurred eyesight.

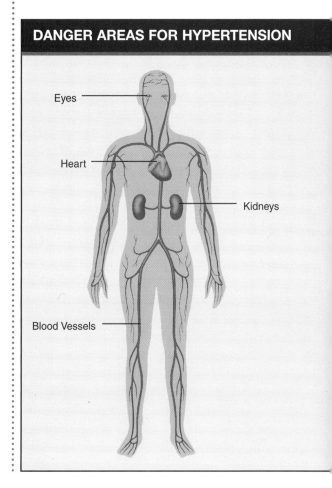

DANGER AREAS FOR HYPERTENSION

Eyes

Heart

Kidneys

Blood Vessels

If your blood pressure is high the doctor will look for signs of organ damage. This involves inspecting the back of your eyes to check for narrowing or thickening of the blood vessels; looking for small hemorrhages inside the eye; listening to your heart to detect any irregularities; checking blood flow in your arteries; and checking the abdomen for signs of kidney enlargement.

EYES
High blood pressure does not seriously damage vision unless it is very high. However, abnormalities in the small blood vessels of the retina can be clearly seen, even in cases of mildly raised blood pressure. They indicate whether blood pressure has been high for some time.

HEART
High blood pressure puts a tremendous strain on the heart. This is partly because less blood is able to reach the heart and also because it forces the heart to work harder to pump blood around the body. Over time, this causes the heart to enlarge and then to weaken as its function deteriorates.

KIDNEYS
High blood pressure damages the tissue and arterioles in the kidneys, causing them to work less efficiently.

BLOOD VESSELS
Untreated high blood pressure causes the blood vessels to narrow and harden and speeds up the development of atherosclerosis, the medical term for thickening of the blood vessel walls, which is linked to heart disease.

1

YOU REALLY NEED TO KNOW

◆ Blood pressure is known as "the silent killer" because usually it causes no symptoms.

◆ If blood pressure remains high without treatment it can cause a lot of damage.

◆ Blood flow becomes sluggish and the blood becomes thicker and clots more easily.

◆ Prompt treatment reduces the risk of developing serious medical problems.

Effects on the body

Related medical conditions

SELF-HELP

✓ Report unusual symptoms, such as breathlessness, wheezing, dizziness, or loss of memory, to your doctor.

✗ Do not miss regular blood pressure and medical check-ups after the age of 40.

Because of the damage it can do to the heart and blood vessels, high blood pressure, if left untreated, can cause a number of medical problems, many of them serious or potentially fatal. Some of these conditions could be avoided simply by having regular blood pressure checks and appropriate treatment.

Heart failure

The effort of pumping out blood at high pressure puts the heart under stress. Over time, in order to cope with the strain, the heart enlarges. Eventually it begins to fail and the blood supply to the rest of the body decreases. As the condition progresses, symptoms include weakness and fatigue. Later, due to the enlargement of the heart, fluid gathers in the lungs and lower limbs causing a cough, breathlessness, swollen feet and ankles.

Kidney failure

Damage to the arterioles obstructs the flow of blood to the kidneys. Eventually the efficiency of kidney function is affected, and they are unable to do the essential job of disposing of waste products, including drugs and alcohol. In the early stages symptoms include nausea, loss of appetite, and fatigue.

Poor eyesight

High blood pressure damages the blood vessels in the eyes. This may, in fact, be the first visible clue to the effect high blood pressure is having on other organs. The doctor can see the damage by examining the back of your eye with an instrument called an ophthalmoscope. Extremely high blood pressure can cause hypertensive retinopathy which can lead to blurred vision and blindness.

Stroke

People with high blood pressure are up to seven times more likely to have a stroke. It is estimated that four out of ten people who die of a stroke could have been saved by having regular blood pressure checks and treatment.

A stroke (sometimes called a brain attack) occurs when the blood supply to the brain is interrupted, usually by a blood clot. Sometimes a stroke occurs when high blood pressure has caused a weak spot in the wall of one of the smaller arteries, which bursts. In either case, the affected part of the brain dies, resulting in speech difficulties, loss of vision, and paralysis.

Transient ischemic attack (TIA)

High blood pressure can also cause a transient ischemic attack (TIA), a ministroke, which may cause temporary eyesight disturbances, dizziness, and changes in sensation. Although the person returns to normal afterward he or she is more at risk of a true stroke.

Symptoms come on suddenly but are always followed by full recovery. If you suspect that you may have had a TIA, report it to your doctor so that treatment can be prescribed to avert a full stroke.

Dementia

Sometimes a series of "little" strokes, which are not severe but produce sudden physical weakness and double vision, gradually damage the brain tissue. If they continue over a long period, the person may become forgetful and confused. Doctors call this multi-infarct dementia (MID) which may sometimes be confused with Alzheimer's disease. However, in MID, drug treatment can slow deterioration.

1

YOU REALLY NEED TO KNOW

◆ Regular blood pressure checks help your doctor monitor your general state of health.

◆ The entire vascular system is at risk if high blood pressure is left untreated.

◆ When the arteries thicken (called atherosclerosis) it can lead to coronary artery disease, heart attacks, and peripheral vascular disease.

Related medical conditions

Related medical conditions

DOs AND DON'Ts

✓ If you have high blood pressure, take symptoms such as chest pain seriously and see your doctor.

✗ Don't be fatalistic about high blood pressure—if it is kept under control you will not become ill because of it.

Coronary artery disease

If the coronary arteries supplying the heart become hard and inelastic, narrow and thickened as a result of high BP, not enough blood gets to the heart. Symptoms can include pain, a feeling of pressure or suffocation in the chest, known as angina, a heart attack, or death.

Heart attack

If a coronary artery narrows so much that blood is unable to get through to the heart, or if an artery is blocked by a clot becoming lodged in the narrowed arteries, part of the heart is starved of blood and dies. This is a heart attack.

Peripheral vascular disease

When the blood vessels supplying the legs are damaged, insufficient blood reaches the fingers and toes. This in turn can lead to pain in the legs, especially on walking. Peripheral vascular disease may lead to leg ulcers and even gangrene caused by the loss of the blood supply to the feet. This condition is also linked to smoking and diabetes.

HOW THE ARTERIES BECOME THICKENED

Arteries have three layers: a smooth inner lining, a muscular layer, and a fibrous outer layer. The lining becomes thickened by patches of plaque, reducing the space available for the flow of blood.

NORMAL ARTERY

THICKENED ARTERY

WHAT DOES IT MEAN?

ANGINA

Chest pain or pressure in the chest felt on exertion. It is caused by insufficient blood reaching the heart. Angina may also be felt as pain in the arms or a choking sensation in the neck and throat.

DEMENTIA

Decline in mental ability causing forgetfulness, confusion, and mood swings. It can be caused by narrowed or blocked arteries in the brain. Treatment of high blood pressure may slow deterioration.

GANGRENE

Death of tissue, caused by loss of blood supply, for example as a result of acute blockage of the arteries.

ISCHEMIA

Insufficient supply of blood to an organ or tissue. A transient ischemic attack (TIA) occurs when the brain is temporarily starved of blood because of blockage of the arteries supplying the brain. It can cause dizziness and visual disturbances. Ischemic heart disease (IHD) is caused by blockage of the coronary arteries.

VASCULAR

A term meaning "of the blood vessels." Peripheral vascular disease is disease in blood vessels far from the heart—in the legs or feet, for example. Like angina, it is caused by an insufficient blood supply to the affected area.

YOU REALLY NEED TO KNOW

◆ Regular blood pressure checks can ensure you get treatment to prevent serious problems from developing.

◆ No matter how severe your high blood pressure is, if it is controlled by treatment and/or lifestyle measures, you have an excellent chance of living a long and healthy life.

Related medical conditions

Chapter

2

TREATMENT &
SELF-HELP

Finding the right treatment

DOs AND DON'Ts

✓ Once you have started treatment, you must return to the doctor for regular blood pressure checks.

✗ It is important that you don't just stop taking your medication. If you are not happy, talk to your doctor about it.

There is a wide range of drugs that your doctor can prescribe to bring your blood pressure down. The aim is to find the particular drug or combination of drugs that will lower your blood pressure to a safe level (ideally to or below 140/85) and prevent problems. The doctor will tailor treatment to you as an individual, so do not be surprised if you find that you are taking completely different drugs from someone else with the same condition.

Why it may take some time

Finding the right drug or combination of drugs may involve a certain amount of trial and error, so be prepared to be patient and to persevere. You will usually be prescribed a low dose of a drug to start with to allow your system to adjust to it and the lower blood pressure. This makes it less likely that you will experience adverse side-effects.

You will be asked to return for regular check-ups to measure the effectiveness of the drug or drugs prescribed. Depending on the results, the doctor may increase your dose or prescribe an additional drug. It is common today to use combination therapy, in which low doses of more than one drug are combined in a single tablet. This is often more effective in controlling blood pressure and produces fewer side-effects than a high dose of a single drug.

Tailoring your medication

Your doctor will tailor your treatment specifically to your needs, selecting the drugs that will deal best with the effects of raised blood pressure on your body. He or she might suggest you keep a diary to note down any side-effects, when they occurred, and what they were.

TYPES OF DRUGS

There are different categories of drugs used to bring high blood pressure within a normal range and they work in three different ways.

DIURETICS

These drugs reduce the amount of fluid in the body by increasing urine flow. Reducing body fluid means that there is less for the heart to pump around the body.

BETA-BLOCKERS

Drugs in this category reduce the heart's workload by preventing the stimulating effects of stress, slowing the heartbeat, and reducing its force. This makes it easier for the heart to pump blood around the body.

OTHERS

These act on the widening and narrowing of the blood vessels. The group includes ACE inhibitors, which block the formation of the hormone angiotensin that causes the blood vessels to narrow; angiotensin II inhibitors, which block the effect of angiotensin; calcium channel blockers, which relax the blood vessels; and alpha-blockers, which, also relax the blood vessels.

Drug treatment for hypertension is not short term. It may be necessary for some years or for the rest of your life, but controlling the condition is likely to give you more years of good health.

YOU REALLY NEED TO KNOW

◆ Finding the correct treatment may take some time and you may have to be patient.

◆ Combination therapy—taking two types of drugs in a single tablet—is often extremely successful and produces fewer side-effects.

◆ Different kinds of blood-pressure-lowering drugs work on the body in different ways.

Finding the right treatment

Medication charts

The charts on this and the following pages show some of the various drugs that may be prescribed and explain how they work and what side-effects they may have. The list is not comprehensive because the range of drugs is wide.

DRUGS USED TO TREAT HIGH BP

DRUG	HOW THEY WORK
DIURETICS ("WATER PILLS" AND POTASSIUM SPARING AGENTS)	Work on kidneys to increase output of urine and reduce volume of circulating blood. (Unlikely to be the main medium of action in the long term.)
BETA-BLOCKERS	Block the action of stress hormones produced by the body that make the heart beat faster, thus slowing the heart rate and reducing the work that the heart has to do. This reduces the amount of oxygen the heart needs and improves its ability to cope with physical exertion.

POSSIBLE SIDE EFFECTS	GENERIC NAMES
Loss of appetite	amiloride
Stomach upsets	bumetanide
Dehydration	chlorthalidone
Impotence	frusemide
High cholesterol and	hydrochlorothiazide
calcium levels	indapamide
Allergic reactions	metolazone
Increased uric acid	spironolactone
Raised blood sugar	torasemide
Muscle weakness	triamterene
Menstrual irregularities	

POSSIBLE SIDE EFFECTS	GENERIC NAMES
Light-headedness	acebutolol
Pins and needles	atenolol
Cold fingers and toes	betaxolol
Upset stomach	bisoprolol
Depression, fatigue	carteolol
Nightmares	esmolol
Wheezing	metoprolol
Drowsiness, lethargy	nadolol
Weakness	penbutolol
Visual disturbances	pindolol
Impotence	propranolol
Elevated blood sugar	timolol
Insomnia	
Low blood sugar	

YOU REALLY NEED TO KNOW

◆ Diuretics and beta-blockers used to be the first line treatment for high blood pressure, but are less frequently prescribed today.

◆ Different people respond to drugs in different ways.

◆ Beta-blockers should never be stopped abruptly. The dose should be gradually reduced over several weeks.

Medication charts

Medication charts

The drugs on this medication chart all act by affecting the mechanism by which the arteries widen and narrow. Widening the arteries allows more blood through so it is an effective way of lowering blood pressure.

DRUGS USED TO TREAT HIGH BP

DRUG	HOW THEY WORK
ACE INHIBITORS (ANGIOTENSIN-CONVERTING ENZYME INHIBITORS)	Block formation of the hormone angiotensin II, which itself causes the blood vessels to narrow. The action of this drug improves blood flow and therefore reduces the amount of work the heart has to do. More salt and water are lost in urine as well.
CALCIUM CHANNEL BLOCKERS (CALCIUM ANTAGONISTS)	Reduce the amount of calcium in the muscular artery walls, relax muscles and cause arteries to widen. This leads to a drop in blood pressure. It also reduces the workload of the heart and cuts down its oxygen needs.

POSSIBLE SIDE EFFECTS	GENERIC NAMES
Dry cough	benazepril
Dizziness on sitting or	captopril
standing up (postural	cilazapril
hypotension)	enalapril
General dizziness	fosinopril
Rash	lisinopril
Allergic reactions	moexipril
Loss of taste	perindopril
Swelling	quinapril
High potassium	ramipril
	trandolapril
Flushing	amlodipine
Headache	diltiazem
Swollen ankles	felodipine
Dizziness	isradepine
Slow or fast heartbeat	nicardipine
Rare side-effects	nifedipine
Fatigue	nisoldipine
Nausea, heartburn	verapamil
Palpitations	
Drowsiness	
Insomnia	
Upset stomach	
Rashes	
Ringing in the ears	
Thickened gums	
Constipation	

YOU REALLY NEED TO KNOW

◆ ACE inhibitors and calcium channel blockers taken in combination seem to have a protective effect on organs such as the kidneys.

◆ Calcium channel blockers appear to be especially effective in lowering blood pressure for African, African-Caribbean, and older people.

Medication charts

Medication charts

The drugs on this medication chart all work by blocking the action of different hormones involved in the widening and narrowing of the arteries.

DRUGS USED TO TREAT HIGH BP

TYPE OF DRUG	HOW THEY WORK
ANGIOTENSIN II ANTAGONISTS	Block the hormone angiotensin II, which narrows the blood vessels in the kidneys, adrenal glands, heart, brain, and sympathetic nervous system.
ALPHA-BLOCKERS ALPHA-BETA BLOCKERS	Alpha-blockers block effects of stress hormones in the arteries, causing the arteries to widen and reducing resistance to the flow of blood. Alpha-beta blockers slow heartbeat so less blood is pumped through the system.
ALPHA-AGONISTS	Work to trick the brain into thinking there is enough stress hormone in the bloodstream. This leads to blood vessels widening in the heart and kidneys.

POSSIBLE SIDE-EFFECTS	GENERIC NAMES
Dizziness	losartan
Muscle cramps	
Back and leg pain	
Insomnia	
Nasal congestion	
High potassium	
Dizziness on standing	doxazosin
(postural hypotension)	prazosin
Vertigo	terazosin
Nausea, headache	labetalol
Lack of energy	
Palpitations	
Passing urine more often	
Fluid retention and edema	
Fainting	
Dry mouth	clonidine*
Fatigue, Lethargy	guanfacine
Impotence	methyldopa
Rare side-effects:	
High fever	*Suddenly stopping this
Liver damage	can lead to a crisis of
	high BP.

YOU REALLY NEED TO KNOW

◆ Alpha-blockers are especially useful for people with diabetes and kidney damage.

◆ Because alpha-blockers help relax the bladder, they may help men with prostate problems but can cause urinary incontinence in women.

Medication charts

Taking your medication

✓ Make sure you know what your medication is for and how you should take it.

✓ Try to get into a routine that makes it easy to remember when to take your drugs.

✗ Even if you feel well do not stop taking your medication. Make an appointment to see your doctor or nurse to discuss it.

For drug treatment of high blood pressure to be effective, it is important that you fully understand your doctor's instructions and follow them carefully.

What your doctor should tell you

Before leaving the doctor's office, make sure you understand exactly what the drug has been prescribed for and what side-effects you can expect. Ask your

YOUR MEDICATION ROUTINE

If you find it difficult to keep track of what you have taken and when, and especially if you have to take several different types of drugs, you may find it useful to get a special drug dispenser. These are designed to help you organize your drugs and remember when to take them. Always check the label for the expiration date of your drugs, and discard any you have not used by this date.

QUESTIONS TO ASK THE DOCTOR

◆ When should I take the drug?

◆ What can I eat or drink when I take the drug?

◆ Should I take the drug with a meal?

◆ Are there any other drugs I cannot take with this drug?

◆ What should I do if I run out of the drug?

◆ What should I do if I forget to take a dose?

doctor how many times a day you need to take the drug, and when and how it should be taken. Most tablets or capsules are best taken with fluid or they might lodge in your throat, which can delay absorption.

When you pick up the prescription, ask the pharmacist if there are any special instructions, though these should be written on the bottle or in the accompanying leaflet.

Follow-up

Your doctor should tell you how often you will have to return to the office for check-ups. You are likely to have to go for more frequent check-ups at first until he or she is satisfied that the right prescription for you has been found. Once the doctor is satisfied that the medication is working with as few side-effects as possible, the number of visits you have to make to the office will decrease.

If you are in doubt about any drug that you have been prescribed, discuss your concerns with your doctor or pharmacist.

YOU REALLY NEED TO KNOW

◆ You may need frequent check-ups until your doctor is satisfied that your drug regime is working.

◆ You may find it helpful to use a special medication dispenser to keep track of when to take your drugs.

◆ Ask the doctor or pharmacist if there are any special instructions connected to taking your drugs.

Taking your medication

Dealing with side-effects

✓ Always report any side-effects you experience to the doctor.

✓ Write down what happened, when it occurred, and how severe it was.

✗ Don't forget to ask if the medication will clash with drugs you may be taking for another condition.

All drugs have side-effects as well as benefits. For example, if you are prescribed a diuretic you will usually find you need to pass urine more often, especially when you first start taking the drug.

It is a good idea to know what side-effects are likely so that if you do develop any of them you can report them to your doctor. The good news is that, with new developments in drugs, the likelihood of experiencing side-effects is becoming smaller. The side-effects listed on the charts on pages 32–37 are those that are commonly linked to the various medications outlined. When listed in this way, they can seem discouraging, but you should bear in mind that many side-effects are mild and wear off once your body has gotten used to the drug.

Weigh the benefits

If you think you are experiencing a side-effect it is vitally important that you do not suddenly stop taking the drug that you believe may be the cause. Instead, make an appointment to see your doctor as soon as possible so you can discuss it. The doctor will weigh the benefits of the drug against the disadvantage of any side-effects and may change the dosage or prescribe a different drug. Try to be patient. It may take a while to find the precise dosage or drug that is best for you.

Finding ways to cope

Some side-effects are more of a nuisance than anything else, and you may be able to get around them with a few self-help measures. If lack of energy is a problem, for example, you could try pacing yourself, paying attention to your eating habits and adding some daily exercise to help improve your energy levels.

Other side-effects ease off after a short period so you may need to deal with it until they do. Your doctor can advise you on how long this should take. If the side-effect does not disappear within a reasonable period, he or she will usually be able to prescribe another drug.

If this isn't possible you may have to accept that putting up with a few minor side-effects is part of getting healthy. It can be hard to see why you need to continue taking a drug that is causing you to feel ill and it will help to keep in mind the greater health benefits of controlling your blood pressure.

Work as a team

It is important to establish a trusting relationship with your doctor and work with him or her to discover your ideal medication regime. You should always feel free to ask questions and it will help if you make your appointments for less busy times so there is time to talk.

Regular sessions with your doctor are part of being treated for high blood pressure. Assessing how the drugs are working and your response to them will involve both of you as a team.

YOU REALLY NEED TO KNOW

◆ It may take some time for your body to get used to the drug or drugs prescribed.

◆ Some side-effects are merely a nuisance, others are more troublesome.

◆ When you report any side effects you experience to the doctor, it may not always be possible to change your prescription.

Dealing with side-effects

Treatment with aspirin

FACTS

Aspirin has a long history of treating headaches and other aches and pains caused by inflammation.

In small doses aspirin works on platelets in the blood to prevent clots from forming.

Aspirin affects the production of hormone-like substances called prostaglandins that can trigger pain, inflammation, or clotting.

Aspirin is often prescribed for people with controlled high blood pressure. It is not used for its pain relieving qualities, but helps reduce the risk of heart attacks and other cardiovascular complications.

Strokes and heart attacks

Most people who have had a stroke, ministrokes (TIAs) or heart attack will be prescribed a baby aspirin to help protect against a repeat of the problem. Baby aspirin is one 81 mg tablet daily, about a quarter of a standard aspirin tablet.

Aspirin does not act directly on the blood pressure. Instead it helps to lower the risk of blood clots forming by reducing the stickiness of platelets, special blood cells that are involved in the clotting process. If a clot forms in the arteries leading to the brain this can cause a stroke or TIA, while a clot in the coronary arteries can cause a heart attack.

HOT TREATMENT

Aspirin is derived from willow bark, and its pain relieving and anti-inflammatory effects have been recognized for a century. However, it is only relatively recently that its anti-clotting properties have been put to use in the treatment of heart disease. An international study, known as the Hypertension Optimal Treatment (HOT) trial found that combining a small dose of aspirin with blood-pressure-lowering drugs in people with high blood pressure reduced the risk of heart attacks by as much as 36 percent.

PLATELETS AND BLOOD VESSELS

Platelets are the smallest blood cells and they play an important role in clotting. Normally, clotting is a useful function. If you get a cut, for example, clotting stops you from bleeding to death and seals the area to prevent infection from entering.

Problems arise, however, inside the body when platelets come into contact with damaged areas on the blood vessel walls (which may have been caused by prolonged and untreated high BP). The blood flow becomes more turbulent, the clotting process is triggered, leading to unwanted blood clots, or thrombi, which are involved in thrombosis, the medical word for abnormal clot formation. If a thrombus forms in a blood vessel supplying the heart or the brain, it can cause a heart attack or stroke.

Preventive action

Aspirin is known medically as an anti-platelet drug. By working chemically on the platelets, a type of red blood cell involved in the process of clotting, aspirin makes blood clots more slippery so they do not lodge in the blood vessels and cause a stroke or heart attack.

Aspirin is sometimes prescribed for people who have angina, which is pain caused by heart disease. Other anti-platelet drugs may be prescribed instead of or as well as aspirin. You should never, however, take aspirin in this way unless under medical supervision.

After a stroke or heart attack, the risk of another is greatest in the next few months, so the sooner preventive treatment is begun the better.

YOU REALLY NEED TO KNOW

◆ Aspirin is prescribed routinely for people who have had a stroke or a heart attack and often for someone who has had a ministroke (TIA).

◆ Aspirin does not treat high blood pressure directly.

◆ People with diabetes have to be careful as large amounts of aspirin can alter blood glucose levels. However, a dose given for high blood pressure is always very small.

Treatment with aspirin

Will I always need medication?

Medication to lower blood pressure can reduce the risk of stroke by 35–40 per cent.

Taking medication to lower blood pressure can reduce the likelihood of developing heart disease by 20–25 per cent.

Research shows that medication to lower blood pressure can dramatically cut your risk of having a stroke and developing heart disease, so it really is well worth continuing to take it.

If you are prescribed drugs to control your blood pressure, you will probably have to take them for the rest of your life. It can be difficult to accept this, especially if you feel perfectly well or if you are experiencing troublesome side-effects.

In a minority of cases it may be possible to gradually stop medication. But if you do it against your doctor's advice your risk of developing serious complications such as heart attack or stroke will rise dramatically. Your blood pressure may become harder to control and you could end up taking even more drugs.

What if I improve my lifestyle?

Making diet and lifestyle changes (see Chapter 3) is one of the most important things you can do to help lower your blood pressure. Research has proved that a combination of lifestyle measures and drug treatment lowers blood pressure in over eight out of ten sufferers and dramatically reduces the risk of complications.

However, lifestyle changes alone will be enough in only a very few cases. If your high blood pressure was mild and you only needed minimal medication, you may be able to control your blood pressure sufficiently in this way. Nevertheless, about half of all people who stop taking drugs to lower their blood pressure have to start taking them again at a later date.

If your doctor does consider your blood pressure to be sufficiently well controlled for you to be able to stop taking medication you will still need regular check-ups.

ROUTINE CHECK-UPS

Once you are settled on your medication and your blood pressure is under control, you will have to return to the doctor's office regularly to have your blood pressure checked. These routine checks are often performed by the nurse rather than the doctor.

◆ You will usually need to have your blood pressure checked about four times a year once it has stabilized.

◆ It is vital that you attend your check-ups to make sure that your blood pressure remains under control.

◆ The doctor may recommend other checks from time to time, perhaps blood tests and EKGs to make sure that your heart, blood vessels, and kidneys are healthy.

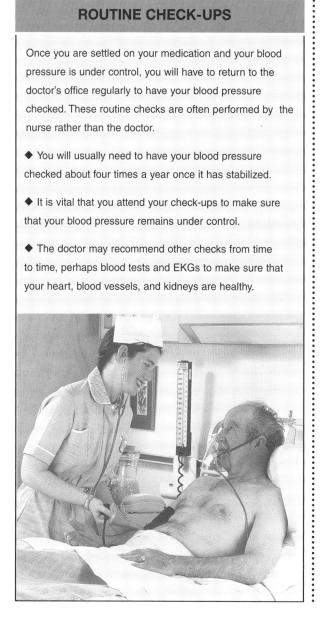

2

**YOU REALLY
NEED TO KNOW**

◆ Only occasionally can lifestyle measures lower blood pressure sufficiently for you to stop taking medication.

◆ If you stop taking medication without your doctor's advice your blood pressure may rise dangerously and become harder to control.

Will I always need medication?

Chapter

DAY-TO-DAY LIFESTYLE

Weight control

SELF-HELP

✓ Diet or join a gym with a friend to help increase your motivation.

✗ Avoid crash diets and miracle solutions. Instead aim to lose weight gradually—it is more likely to stay off that way.

Excess weight increases the work your heart has to do in pumping blood around your body. If you are overweight you are also more likely to have high cholesterol and to develop diabetes—both of which increase your risk of having heart disease or a stroke. These risks are even greater in women than in men. Weight control is believed by many experts to be an important factor in reducing the risk of high blood pressure.

Losing weight will help to lower your blood pressure and reduce your risk of having a stroke, heart attack, or other serious illnesses. Research has found that for every two pounds you lose your blood pressure will fall by one millimeter of mercury. If your blood pressure is only slightly raised, shedding excess pounds may return it to normal without the need for medication.

WHY A HEALTHY DIET IS THE BEST WEIGHT-LOSS DIET

The best way to lose weight is gradually. On a low-calorie diet your body, thinking it is starved of food, raids the muscles for the fuel stored there (this is the first weight you lose) and this saps your energy. Your metabolism slows down. On a healthy diet, a steady reduction in weight occurs as stored fat is burned, so your muscle increases and you also have a lot more energy.

Energy

Muscle

Fat

Weight

◾ Calorie-controlled diet   ◾ Healthy diet

EFFECTIVE WEIGHT LOSS

◆ Aim to lose weight slowly—one to two pounds a week.

◆ The best way to lose weight is to cut down on fatty and sugary foods and eat more fresh fruit and vegetables.

◆ Weight-loss diets work better if combined with exercise.

How to lose weight

The food you eat provides your body with energy. Ideally, you should not take in any more than your body can use. If you do consume more, you will put on weight because the body turns the excess to fat, which it stores.

To lose weight you need to put into your mouth fewer calories than you burn up (a calorie is simply a unit of energy). The best way to lose weight is to eat less and burn up more calories through increasing the amount of physical activity you do.

If your doctor feels you need to lose weight, you may be given a diet plan to follow. If you have more than a few pounds to lose, you may be referred to a dietician who can advise you on a sensible, healthy eating plan.

Get support

Some people find it hard to persevere with a long-term weight-loss program. If you are one of them it may help to join Weight Watchers or a similar program where you will get advice on losing weight and support from other people with a common goal. If you are struggling to maintain a healthy eating regime, try to keep in mind how much better you will feel once you have lost weight.

YOU REALLY NEED TO KNOW

◆ Excess weight forces your heart to work harder and increases your risk of heart disease, stroke and diabetes.

◆ Every pound of weight you lose has a direct effect on lowering your blood pressure.

◆ The best way to lose weight is through a combination of diet and exercise.

Weight control

What to eat and drink

SELF-HELP

Aim to eat at least five servings of fruit and vegetables a day.

Avoid eating processed foods and do not add salt to your food at the table. Try using herbs, spices, and lemon to season foods instead.

Sea salt, rock salt, and natural salt are as bad for elevated blood pressure as ordinary table or cooking salt.

What you eat and drink has a major effect on your blood pressure. In particular, reducing the amount of salt (sodium chloride) and fatty foods and increasing the amount of fruit and vegetables you eat can help lower your blood pressure and prevent high blood pressure from developing.

Bypass the salt

An excess of salt in the diet can increase blood pressure. Processed foods such as hamburgers, sausages, salted snacks, canned vegetables and meats, bouillon cubes, sauces, and TV dinners contain a lot of salt, so cut down on these and eat more fresh fruit, vegetables, meat, and fish instead. When buying prepared foods, check the labels and choose those labeled "low sodium" or "unsalted." Avoid adding salt to your food when you cook and at the table. "Low salt," which is a third sodium chloride and two thirds potassium chloride, is available as a healthier alternative.

If you persevere with a low-salt diet, you will gradually find that you lose your taste for it after a month or so. If you really can't do without it, there are salt substitutes available containing little or no sodium. They should be used with care if you are taking diuretics or your kidneys are not working well. Ask your doctor to advise you.

Cut down on fat

Doctors and scientists do not yet know whether eating a high-fat diet raises blood pressure. However, a high fat intake (especially the saturated fat in animal products) can raise blood cholesterol levels, which in turn increases the risk of heart disease. In particular, avoid fatty meat such as chicken skin, sausages and burgers, and dairy products like whole milk, cream, and cheese.

WHAT DOES IT MEAN?

ANTI-OXIDANTS

Natural chemicals in fruit and vegetables that help to protect the body's cells against damage from free radicals.

CHOLESTEROL

A natural waxy substance made by the liver and essential for cells. In some people an excess builds up in the blood vessels and contributes to the thickening (plaque formation) of the arteries linked to heart disease and stroke.

FREE RADICALS

Rogue molecules produced in the body by normal processes such as breathing and digestion. Their chemical action on cells causes damage that is thought to be an important factor in heart disease and stroke.

SATURATED FAT

The type of fat found in meat, poultry (especially the skin), milk, butter, cream, cheese, and many purchased baked goods (pastry, cookies). It solidifies at room temperature.

SODIUM CHLORIDE

The chemical name for salt.

More fruit and vegetables

Fresh fruit and vegetables contain chemicals called anti-oxidants that help mop up other chemicals called free radicals, which cause damage to blood vessels. Fruit and vegetables also contain the mineral potassium, which may also lower blood pressure. Eat vegetables raw, when possible, and never overcook them.

YOU REALLY NEED TO KNOW

◆ Read the list of ingredients on store-bought foods. Avoid any in which salt, sugar, or fat are high on the list.

◆ Eating fewer fatty foods helps reduce cholesterol levels and lowers the risk of heart disease.

◆ Eating a wide variety of fruit and vegetables every day can help protect against high blood pressure.

What to eat and drink

Moderate drinking

SELF-HELP

Try to drink alcohol only with food or intersperse drinks with water.

Ask your doctor about drinking if you have had a stroke or heart attack.

Keep to sensible drinking levels and aim to have one or two alcohol-free days every week.

Be aware of the alcohol content of what you are drinking. Some canned and bottled beers are twice as strong as others.

Don't binge. You should never drink all your weekly alcohol allowance at once.

While a small amount of alcohol is believed by some experts to help protect against heart disease, regularly drinking too much can raise your blood pressure and increase your chance of having a stroke. Drinking a lot all at once (binging) is especially harmful. In fact, it can increase your risk of having a stroke or cerebral hemorrhage fivefold. This is because it can cause blood pressure to rise steeply, which in turn increases the risk of a blood vessel bursting and bleeding into your brain.

It is also worth bearing in mind, if you are trying to lose weight, that alcoholic drinks can be measured in calories—which may be another good reason to keep your consumption moderate.

KNOW YOUR ALCOHOL UNITS

One unit of alcohol is equivalent to one small drink. That is about a small glass (4 ounces) of wine, a jigger of alcohol or a glass (8 ounces) of weak beer or lager. With stronger beers or wines, a unit may be significantly more. For example, a small glass of sherry contains one and a half units of alcohol.

Women are advised to keep alcohol intake to two units of drink a day—no more than 14 a week. Men should keep alcohol intake to no more than four units a day—no more than 21 a week.

Learn to keep track of what you are drinking so that you know when you have had enough.

Beware, especially in restaurants—it is all too easy to just keep filling your glass to the top and to go over your limit without really being aware of it.

Sensible drinking

Sticking to sensible drinking levels and avoiding binges can help to reduce your blood pressure and lower your risk of having a heart attack or stroke. Follow the recommendations for men and women (below), and spread your drinking through the week rather than drinking your weekly allowance on one or two days. Aim to have one or two alcohol-free days every week.

Try to drink slowly, sipping your drink and fully appreciating the flavor, rather than just knocking it back. Take the edge off your thirst with a soft drink first so that you do not gulp down your drink. Also try to intersperse alcohol with soft drinks.

Maximum weekly consumption for women = 14 units

Maximum weekly consumption for men = 21 units

YOU REALLY NEED TO KNOW

◆ Binging on alcohol can cause blood pressure to rise to a very high level, increasing the risk of a stroke.

◆ Regularly drinking to excess can also raise blood pressure and may cause liver damage.

◆ Drinking a small quantity on several days a week is better than drinking a much larger quantity on any given day.

Moderate drinking

Enjoying exercise

DOs AND DON'Ts

✓ Aim to do something active most days—choose a form of exercise or activity that you enjoy.

✓ Start slowly and build up gradually so you won't become bored or exhausted.

✗ Don't overdo it. Avoid very competitive or vigorous forms of sports, such as squash or weight training.

✗ Don't go for the "burn." Exercise does not have to hurt to do you good, and you risk injury, which will disrupt your exercise program.

Lack of physical activity can increase your blood pressure, and lead to weight gain. Getting regular exercise can lower your blood pressure and will also help you to control your weight. It will make you look and feel better, and has even been found to help relieve depression.

How much exercise?

If you have not exercised recently and have been diagnosed with high blood pressure (especially if you are taking medication) or have had a stroke or heart attack, you should check with your doctor before embarking on an exercise program. You could seek the help of a local

HOW EXERCISE HELPS

Regular aerobic exercise, the kind that uses oxygen and makes you feel out of breath, helps strengthen your heart and improves its ability to pump blood, thereby reducing its overall workload. Aerobic exercise also helps to burn fat.

gym to help you achieve 30 minutes of moderate physical activity on at least five days a week. If this seems daunting, or if you are short of time, it is not necessary to do the 30 minutes at once—you could break it into three ten-minute sessions, for example.

What kind of exercise?

Any physical activity will do, from a brisk walk to gardening or housework, as long as you break a sweat and are slightly out of breath. If you can't manage that at first, do whatever you can and build up gradually.

One way to fulfill your exercise quota could be simply to incorporate more activity into your daily life—by walking rather than taking a bus, for example, or climbing the stairs rather than taking an escalator or elevator. This kind of approach is particularly useful for people who feel they don't have time to exercise. Practically the only thing to avoid if you have high blood pressure is competitive or vigorous exercise such as marathon running, squash, sit-ups, or weight training.

Keeping it up

It is important to keep up your exercise program, even if your blood pressure goes down. If you stop, your blood pressure may return to its previous level. If you find it hard to stay motivated, you may find it helps to exercise with a friend. Exercise is more enjoyable if you have company, and you are less likely to be tempted to skip, say, a swimming session if you've made an arrangement to meet your friend at the pool. You could also vary your activities to add interest—for example, you could go for a walk three days a week and swim, cycle, play badminton or tennis, or do some gardening on the others.

YOU REALLY NEED TO KNOW

◆ Regular exercise can help lower your blood pressure, reduce your weight, and make you look and feel better.

◆ Everyday activities such as walking can form part of an exercise program.

◆ It is important to maintain your exercise program or you will lose the benefits.

Enjoying exercise

Quitting smoking

DOs AND DON'Ts

✓ Start now. The benefits of giving up smoking are immediate and they increase with time.

✗ Don't feel that all is lost if you slip up sometimes. Just congratulate yourself that you have done well so far and keep on trying.

Smoking increases the risk of heart attack, stroke, and other arterial diseases. If you smoke you are at least twice as likely to suffer a stroke as someone who does not smoke, and five times more likely to develop heart disease. It is estimated that 24 percent of deaths from coronary artery disease in men, and 11 percent in women, are due to smoking.

The effects on your body

Every puff you take on a cigarette acts on the blood vessels and causes them to constrict. Over time, smoking causes thickening and narrowing of the arteries and makes your blood more likely to clot—both of which increase your risk of heart disease and having a stroke. What is more, smoking multiplies the dangers of other risk factors such as diabetes and high blood cholesterol levels, especially in women.

There are plenty of aids to help you quit smoking, including patches, chewing gums, and nasal sprays. These work by allowing you gradually to lose your nicotine dependence.

FIVE STEPS TO SUCCESS

◆ Keep in mind the benefits of giving up smoking.

◆ Take it one step at a time.

◆ Ask your doctor about nicotine patches and other aids.

◆ Enlist the support of your family and friends and ask your doctor about help that is available locally.

◆ Avoid situations where you routinely have a cigarette. If you usually have one with a mid-morning coffee, change your routine to break the habit. Go for a walk instead.

The good news is that if you quit, no matter how long you have been a smoker, your risks go down. Giving up smoking will cut your risk of having a stroke in half.

Ways to give it up

Quitting smoking is not always easy but there are lots of things you can do to help yourself. Giving up smoking with a friend or relative can help keep up your motivation and many doctors now run special groups for people wanting to stop smoking. Nicotine chewing gums, nasal sprays, and patches can also help to quell the craving for a cigarette. Ask your doctor about them.

Think about your daily routine, pinpointing the times when you are most likely to light up. Consider what changes you could make. Starting an exercise routine can have a calming effect and improve your motivation. Stress-reduction techniques may also help you to deal with the tension caused by giving up smoking.

YOU REALLY NEED TO KNOW

◆ Smoking has a direct effect on the walls of blood vessels and therefore on blood pressure.

◆ In women, it multiplies the dangers of diabetes and high cholesterol levels.

◆ Over time, smoking contributes to thickening and narrowing of the arteries and makes your blood more likely to clot.

◆ Giving up tobacco and nicotine will bring immediate and long-term benefits.

Quitting smoking

Managing stress

✓ **Put yourself first. Schedule a little time every day to relax.**

✓ **Learn some problem-solving skills so that you feel more in control of stressful situations.**

✗ **Don't waste time worrying about things that you can't change.**

Feeling anxious or tense elevates your blood pressure in the short term because stress causes the release of hormones that narrow your blood vessels and force your heart to beat harder. Even so, doctors are still not sure whether long-term stress is harmful to the blood vessels.

A sense of control

Researchers have discovered that the amount of control people feel they have over their lives can affect physical health. Those who feel more out of control tend to have higher blood pressure and are more likely to experience heart attacks. The results seem to imply that learning to approach life's inevitable ups-and-downs in a practical, constructive way may lower your blood pressure.

Yoga is an excellent way of tackling stress. It teaches breathing techniques that can be used in any situation and improves flexibility, relieving the muscular tension often caused by stress. It is also suitable for people of all ages.

DEALING WITH YOUR WORRIES

If you are a habitual worrier, learning effective ways to deal with problems can help you feel more in control.

◆ Define the problem.

◆ Make a list of possible solutions.

◆ Select the solutions that are most practical.

◆ Enlist any support you need.

◆ Put your plan into action.

◆ Think positively.

Make time to relax

A balance between work, rest, and play is important. Try to build time for relaxation into your daily life. Many busy people feel they don't have time for it, but you will work more productively and efficiently if you are relaxed. Stopping to relax can be a better investment than spending half an hour tackling a problem when you are too tired and stressed to think straight.

Resting your mind

Relaxation does not necessarily mean doing nothing. For example, someone watching television may actually be thinking through their problems. Active pursuits, such as gardening or dancing, can be restful because they take your mind off your problems and help to disperse stress hormones. Studies have also shown that meditation can lower blood pressure while you are doing it.

YOU REALLY NEED TO KNOW

◆ Stress forces the heart to beat harder and elevates blood pressure in the short term.

◆ People who feel they have little control over their lives often have high blood pressure.

◆ It is important to make time for regular relaxation and pursuits that you enjoy.

◆ Physical activity can be relaxing and can reduce stress levels.

Managing stress

Chapter

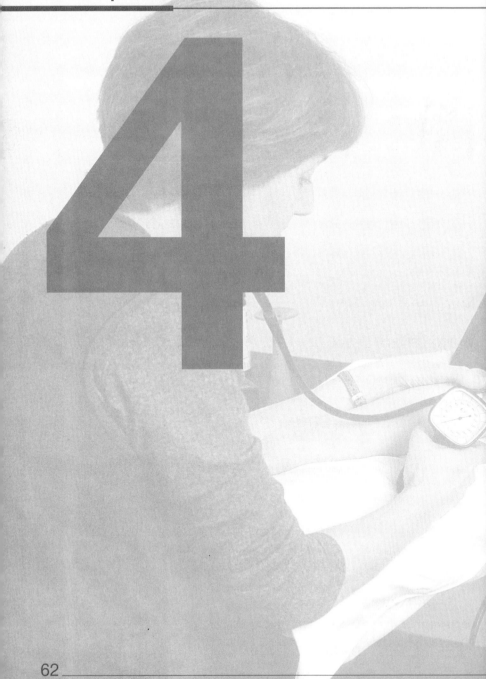

SPECIAL CASES

Pregnancy

DOs AND DON'Ts

✓ It helps to go to bed earlier so that you get at least eight hours' sleep a night.

✗ Try not to worry. Mildly elevated blood pressure will not usually harm your baby.

✗ Don't miss your check-ups and prenatal visits.

Pregnancy causes enormous changes in the amount of blood flowing around the body and in blood pressure. This is partly because the heart beats faster and partly because the hormones of pregnancy cause the blood vessels to relax.

During the first 20 weeks of pregnancy, blood pressure remains the same or lower than before the pregnancy. After this it drops as the blood vessels in the body dilate and the placenta pumps blood to the baby. During the first few months fainting and dizziness can sometimes be a problem due to low blood pressure.

Why your BP is monitored

Blood pressure measurement is one of the routine tests carried out at every prenatal check up. This is because a elevated blood pressure during pregnancy can sometimes be a sign of a serious disease called preeclampsia (see p. 66). Treatment of high blood pressure in pregnancy depends on when it begins. If it occurs after 28 weeks, it may be a sign of preeclampsia and immediate action may have to be taken.

Possible treatment

If you have high blood pressure in early pregnancy it may be that your blood pressure was high before you became pregnant but you were not aware of it.

If your blood pressure is only mildly elevated, the doctor may advise lifestyle measures and rest to help improve the blood supply to the baby. You will have frequent check-ups and the doctor will try to decide whether you need drug treatment.

If your blood pressure is severely elevated you will usually need to be admitted to the hospital for tests to

WHAT DOES IT MEAN?

PLACENTA

An organ that forms in the uterus during pregnancy and to which the growing fetus is attached by the umbilical cord. The placenta is rich in blood vessels through which the fetus receives its blood supply from the mother.

PRENATAL VISITS

Routine medical check-ups during pregnancy to monitor the health of mother and baby. These may take place once a month early in the pregnancy, increasing to once a week toward the end.

YOU REALLY NEED TO KNOW

◆ A pregnant woman has an extra two quarts of blood flowing around her body.

◆ Low blood pressure can be a problem in early pregnancy, causing fainting.

◆ Your blood pressure should be measured at every prenatal visit during pregnancy.

◆ If blood pressure is severely elevated, hospital admission may be needed to check for problems such as kidney disease or diabetes.

check for problems such as kidney disease or diabetes. Your urine will be collected for 24 hours to make sure the problem is not affecting your kidneys and a sonogram will be performed to ensure that your baby is growing properly. Medication to lower blood pressure may be prescribed, though some drugs are unsuitable.

Self-help during pregnancy

If you are found to have elevated blood pressure ask your doctor what is safe for you to do. In general you should try to get as much rest as possible, in the day as well as at night, and avoid any prolonged or vigorous exercise. Eat a sensible diet with plenty of fresh fruit and vegetables, wholegrains, lean meat, chicken, and fish.

Lying on one side when in bed can help improve the blood supply to your baby by reducing pressure on the blood vessels behind your uterus.

Preeclampsia

FACTS

✓ Preeclampsia affects 25 per cent of women during their first pregnancy.

✓ Women who are over 30 are more at risk of developing preeclampsia.

✓ Preeclampsia usually disappears completely within a few weeks of birth.

About one in four women expecting their first baby develops a condition called preeclampsia, which is characterized by high blood pressure. It can also occur in subsequent pregnancies, though this is less common. The condition disappears when the baby is born. The doctor may advise bed rest and possibly drug treatment if this is thought necessary.

What are the symptoms?

A steep rise in blood pressure to 140/90 or more after 28 weeks of pregnancy together with swollen ankles, hands or feet, sudden weight gain, and protein in the urine are signs of preeclampsia. It is not known exactly what causes this condition, but it is thought to be due to an abnormality of the placenta. If it is left untreated, preeclampsia can develop into eclampsia, a dangerous condition that can cause convulsions and threaten the lives of both mother and baby.

If you have preeclampsia you may be admitted to the hospital so that you and your baby can be monitored.

WHEN PREECLAMPSIA IS A RISK

◆ In a first pregnancy.

◆ If you had preeclampsia in a previous pregnancy.

◆ If your mother had it.

◆ If you are expecting twins.

◆ If you have diabetes.

◆ If you are overweight.

WHAT ARE THE DANGER SIGNS?

Contact your doctor immediately if you are in the late stages of pregnancy and experience any of the following signs which can indicate increased blood pressure:

◆ A sudden severe headache.

◆ Visual disturbance.

◆ Abdominal pain.

The only real cure is delivery of the baby. If your blood pressure continues to rise or the baby's growth is being affected, the doctor may decide to deliver your baby early. You will usually be offered epidural anesthesia during labor as this lowers the blood pressure.

Follow-up

In most women their blood pressure comes down after the baby's birth and they experience no further problems. (Preeclampsia is less common in second and subsequent pregnancies.) Sometimes, however, blood pressure stays elevated, and treatment and further tests may be needed.

There is also evidence that some women who have had preeclampsia have a higher risk of developing high blood pressure in later life. For this reason it is a good idea to ask your doctor to check your blood pressure every year if you suffered from preeclampsia during pregnancy. You should know what the risks are of developing it again before trying to have another baby.

YOU REALLY NEED TO KNOW

◆ A sudden rise in blood pressure, swelling, and protein in the urine are signs of preeclampsia.

◆ Preeclampsia is a potentially dangerous condition that only affects pregnant women.

◆ If you have had preeclampsia you may be prone to high blood pressure in later life.

Preeclampsia

The pill and HRT

SELF-HELP

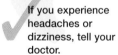

If you experience headaches or dizziness, tell your doctor.

Never miss your check-ups when on the pill or using HRT.

Both oral contraceptives, popularly called the pill, and hormone replacement therapy (HRT) can affect blood pressure. Each has differing amounts of the female sex hormone estrogen, which is thought to be the cause.

Taking contraception

The combined contraceptive pill, which contains estrogen and progestogen, can cause a small rise in blood pressure, which is usually not of any importance. A few women, however, (around 5 percent), experience a rise in diastolic blood pressure to over 90 mm Hg; occasionally there may be a more severe rise. The problem is more likely to occur in women who are over 35, are overweight, smoke, or have a previous history of high blood pressure. Your doctor may recommend low-estrogen or progestogen-only contraception, which is less likely to cause problems.

You may be able to take the pill even if you have high blood pressure, provided you have regular blood pressure checks. Ask your doctor for advice.

At menopause

HRT is prescribed to help with symptoms of menopause caused by reduced estrogen levels, such as hot flashes, vaginal dryness, mood swings, and reduced libido. It is known to protect against the brittle bone disease, osteoporosis, and to be the most effective way of building bone after menopause.

HRT contains estrogen but in much lower doses than the contraceptive pill. HRT does not contribute to elevated BP and has been found to lower the risk of heart attack and stroke, which are much more common in people with high blood pressure.

WHAT DOES IT MEAN?

WORD	DEFINITION
COMBINED ORAL CONTRACEPTIVE PILL	A contraceptive pill containing the two female sex hormones, estrogen and progestogen.
HRT	Hormone replacement therapy, estrogen and progestogen treatment, is prescribed at or after the menopause to counteract symptoms and protect against, or treat, brittle bones.
ESTROGEN	One of the two main female sex hormones. It is thought to be protective against heart disease before menopause.
OSTEOPOROSIS	A disease in which the bones lose density, causing them to become brittle and break more easily. It is most common in women after menopause.
PROGESTOGEN	One of the two major female sex hormones. Progestogen-only contraceptives may be less likely to cause a rise in blood pressure.

YOU REALLY NEED TO KNOW

◆ Some types of oral contraceptives cause a small rise in blood pressure.

◆ You are more likely to experience a rise in blood pressure if you are over 35, overweight, smoke, or have previously had high blood pressure.

◆ HRT is less likely to cause a rise in blood pressure if your blood pressure is normal when you start using it.

◆ If you take the contraceptive pill or HRT, your blood pressure should be checked regularly.

The pill and HRT

Medical conditions

DOs AND DON'Ts

✓ Tell your doctor about any treatments you are taking for asthma or breathing problems if he suggests beta-blockers to control your high blood pressure.

✗ Don't be concerned if you develop a dry cough when taking ACE inhibitors—this is not usually significant.

Some medical conditions can increase the risk of high blood pressure; in others it is inadvisable for certain types of drugs that lower BP to be prescribed.

Diabetes

There are two types of diabetes, a condition in which the the body is unable to use sugar (glucose) in the bloodstream. In Type 1 the body does not produce enough insulin whereas in Type 2 the body does not respond properly to what insulin there is. Until recently the main treatment for diabetes has been to manage blood glucose levels through diet, drugs, or by injecting insulin. However, research shows that controlling blood pressure is just as important. One in every two people with Type 2 diabetes (adult-onset, the most common form) also has high BP, putting them at unusually high risk of heart disease, stroke, blindness and, especially, kidney failure.

In someone with diabetes, the danger level of blood pressure is lower than the commonly accepted 140/85. If you have diabetes your doctor will monitor you closely and may treat you if your BP rises above 130/80.

Arthritis

Arthritis is inflammation causing pain, swelling, and stiffness in the joints. There are many different types. Rheumatoid arthritis is a chronic condition, which causes gradual destruction of the joints and can also affect the heart, lungs, and eyes. It is often treated with non-steroidal anti-inflammatory drugs (NSAIDs) which can make you insensitive to a previously effective BP regimen. Your doctor will need to take both conditions into account when deciding how to treat you.

WHAT DOES IT MEAN?

CHRONIC CONDITION
A disease that goes on for a long time, such as diabetes, as opposed to one that can be treated and disappears.

INSULIN
A hormone produced by the pancreas, which controls levels of glucose in the blood.

PANCREAS
One of the body's glands, which produces the hormone, insulin, needed to control blood glucose. Failure of the pancreas to produce enough insulin is a cause of diabetes.

Chest problems

People with asthma or other diseases causing breathing difficulties should not take beta-blocker drugs, so it is important to remind your doctor if you are being treated for such a condition. A minority of patients stop taking ACE inhibitors because they develop an irritating cough.

Heart disease

If you have angina (chest or arm pain caused by blocked arteries), beta-blockers can help reduce the number of attacks you have. The doctor may prescribe other drugs such as those to lower cholesterol; this is also the case if you have had a heart attack as these drugs will reduce your chance of a further attack. ACE inhibitors and beta-blockers can be especially helpful as they can lower blood pressure as well as reducing the amount of work the heart has to do.

YOU REALLY NEED TO KNOW

◆ If you have diabetes, it is especially important that your blood pressure and blood glucose levels are both controlled.

◆ If you have arthritis, some drugs used to treat it may raise your blood pressure.

◆ It may be inadvisable for anyone with asthma or breathing problems to be prescribed beta-blockers.

Medical conditions

Whom should I tell?

For your own safety, be sure to tell all your medical practitioners about your condition.

Don't neglect to tell relevant insurance companies— otherwise your policies could be invalidated.

Because of the implications for your health, there are a number of people who need to know if you are diagnosed with high blood pressure.

Medical practitioners

You should inform all your medical and paramedical practitioners, such as general or specialist doctors, physical therapist, podiatrist, dentist, ambulance personnel, and anyone else who treats you for a health-related problem.

It is important if you need treatment for any other condition because some drugs may interact with the drugs you are taking to lower your blood pressure.

If you have to see another doctor, either in the office or in the hospital, always make sure he or she knows you are being treated for elevated blood pressure.

If you are pregnant and have been diagnosed with high blood pressure, you should inform your doctor and any other health professionals that you come into contact with.

Complementary practitioners

If you seek help from an alternative or complementary therapist such as a homeopath, acupuncturist, herbalist, aromatherapist, or osteopath, tell them if you have high blood pressure. You should never stop taking any medication prescribed by your doctor on the advice of a complementary or alternative therapist.

Before accepting treatment from a complementary practitioner, check him or her out carefully. Ask about their license, certification, insurance, qualifications and accreditation by regulatory bodies. Steer clear of anyone who promises you a miracle cure. There isn't one.

4

WHAT DOES IT MEAN?

AROMATHERAPY

A complementary therapy that uses essential oils from parts of plants and massage to restore wellbeing.

HERBALISM

A complementary therapy that uses herbs and herbal extracts to treat illness.

HOMEOPATHY

A therapy that involves treating illnesses with greatly diluted doses of the same substance that is thought to cause the illness.

OSTEOPATHY

A therapy that involves massage and manipulation of the bones to treat musculoskeletal pain, particularly of the back and limbs.

PARAMEDICAL

Describes health practitioners who support doctors, such as physical therapists, podiatrists, and ambulance personnel.

The pharmacist

Because certain high blood pressure treatments may interact with other types of medication it is important to tell the pharmacist you are being treated for high blood pressure. This applies whether you are getting a prescription medication or buying over-the-counter products for minor conditions. The pharmacist can be an invaluable source of advice on the possible interactions between one drug type and another.

**YOU REALLY
NEED TO KNOW**

If you are diagnosed with high blood pressure and are being treated with drugs you should inform:

◆ All medical and paramedical practitioners with whom you come into contact.

◆ Your pharmacist.

◆ Your fitness instructor.

◆ Your insurance companies (personal and car).

You may also need to inform:

◆ Your employer.

◆ The department of motor vehicles (DMV) or appropriate vehicle licensing authority.

◆ Your vacation or tour operator.

Whom should I tell?

Whom should I tell?

DOs AND DON'Ts

✓ Do remember to carry your medication for high blood pressure with you at all times.

✗ Don't forget to tell your instructor about your medical condition if you join a gym or fitness class.

Your employer

Elevated blood pressure that is being treated will not usually be a problem at work. However, your employer may need to know about your condition if you have a job—such as roofing—that involves working at a height.

If you have high blood pressure you may not be allowed to join the police, fire service, or armed services. If you already work in one of these jobs, you may be allowed to continue working provided your blood pressure is controlled.

The vehicle licensing authorities

The DMV or your vehicle licensing authority will not usually need to know if you have high blood pressure for an ordinary driver's license. However, if you drive a truck, bus, or other heavy vehicle, special rules apply and you will need to inform them. Whatever kind of license you hold, you will need to inform the driving licensing authority if you have had a stroke or heart attack or if you have diabetes.

Insurance companies

If you are being treated for high blood pressure, you must inform any insurance company with whom you hold a health or life insurance policy—if you do not, the policy may not be valid and when you come to make a claim there may not be a payment.

Also inform your insurance company of any changes in your medical state if you hold certain other types of policy that have a life insurance element. They may also be affected. You should also mention your condition when you take out any insurance policy that covers you for medical treatment—vacation insurance, for example.

You may find that some life insurance companies charge high premiums if you have high blood pressure. It is worth shopping around for the best policy.

Vacation and travel

Having high blood pressure should not prevent you going away on vacation. However, it pays to plan your trip carefully beforehand so you can be free from worries while you are away. As with many other medical conditions, when choosing your destination it is sensible to avoid very remote areas where it might be difficult to obtain medical attention, should you need it.

You may need to tell the tour operator and airline, especially if your high blood pressure is associated with another condition such as heart disease.

Allow yourself plenty of time to pack and prepare for your vacation to avoid undue stress and make sure that you allow plenty of time for the journey. If you are flying for longer than four hours, take your daily aspirin just before you board the plane and drink plenty of water during the flight. Get up and walk around every two hours or so in order to prevent the stagnation of the blood flow through the feet and legs.

Fitness instructors

If you belong to a gym or fitness center or embark on an activity such as an aerobics or yoga class you should inform the instructor that you have high blood pressure and whether you are taking medication for it.

This enables the instructor to make sure that you are not encouraged to do anything that could potentially exacerbate your condition, and ensures that you are insured while on the premises.

YOU REALLY NEED TO KNOW

◆ High blood pressure is not usually a problem at work, unless your job involves working at a height or driving a bus or truck.

◆ You must inform the Department of Motor Vehicles or your vehicle licensing authority if you have had a stroke, a heart attack, or have diabetes.

◆ Vacation insurance which precludes pre-existing conditions will not be acceptable if you are taking medication for elevated blood pressure.

Whom should I tell?

Understanding the jargon

Medicine is full of technical terms and words that can make a condition such as high blood pressure seem more daunting than it really is. Knowing what the terms mean can clarify your condition and enable you to communicate more easily with your doctor.

ACUTE—Used to describe a medical condition that comes on suddenly and lasts for only a limited period of time.

ANTI-HYPERTENSIVE MEDICATION—Range of drugs administered to lower high blood pressure.

AORTA—The body's main artery, which leads from the heart, running down the back of the heart to the abdomen.

ARTERIES—The largest blood vessels in the body; they transport oxygen-rich blood from the heart to the rest of the body.

ARTERIOLES—Blood vessels that branch from the arteries and supply the organs and tissues with blood. Arterioles are smaller than arteries.

ATHEROSCLEROSIS—A disease in which the lining of the artery walls becomes thickened with fatty deposits (such as cholesterol) plus decaying cells and other waste substances.

ARTERIOSCLEROSIS—A disease in which the arterial walls become hard and thickened and lose elasticity. It is commonly called hardening of the arteries.

CARDIOVASCULAR DISEASE—Disease affecting the heart and the blood vessels.

CHRONIC—A disease or medical condition that lasts for a long time.

CIRCULATORY SYSTEM—The heart and the blood vessels, which are responsible for keeping blood flowing around the body.

DIASTOLE—The part of the heartbeat when the heart is at rest.

HYPERTENSION—High blood pressure.

HYPOTENSION—Low blood pressure.

ISCHAEMIA—Insufficient blood supply to an organ or tissue, usually caused by narrowing of the arteries.

PREECLAMPSIA—A disease leading to high blood pressure during late pregnancy.

SPHYGMOMANOMETER—A device used to measure blood pressure, consisting of a cuff, pressure device, and a mercury column in a glass tube from which the measurements are read.

SYSTOLE—The part of the heartbeat when the heart is contracting.

THROMBUS—An abnormal blood clot.

VASCULAR—A term relating to the body's blood vessels.

VEINS—Blood vessels that return deoxygenated blood to the heart.

Useful addresses

**HEART AND STROKE
FOUNDATION OF CANADA**
222 Queen Street
Suite 1402
Ottawa, ON
KIP 5V9
Telephone: (613) 569-4361
Fax (613) 569-3278

**THE CANADIAN HYPERTENSION
SOCIETY**
c/o Department of Pharmacology
Room A329, Chown Building
University of Manitoba
753 McDermot Avenue
Winnipeg, MB
R3E OT6

USEFUL WEBSITES
Health Canada Online:
http://www.hc-sc.gc.ca/

Index

Index

Acknowledgments
Photographs: Simon Fraser/SPL: 8–9, 43;
Saturn Stills/SPL: 15, 19; Eamon Mcnulty/SPL: 30–31;
Light Productions/SPL: 47; Jerome Yeats/SPL: 48–49; Sam Ogden/SPL: 56;
Andrew Sydenham: 58; Laura Wickenden: 60;
Faye Norman/SPL: 62–63; Damien Lovegrove/SPL: 73

Illustrations: Kuo Kang Chen: 24, 28; Martin Laurie: 10, 14, 22, 50, 55